AF221157

Ayurvedic Diet Cookbook

Ayurvedic Recipes for Pacifying Doshas and Promoting Healthy Weight Loss

Anand Gupta

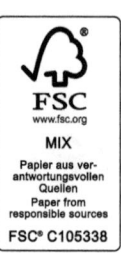

Bibliografische Information der Deutschen Nationalbibliothek:

Die Deutsche Nationalbibliothek verzeichnet diese Publikation in der Deutschen Nationalbibliografie; detaillierte bibliografische Daten sind im Internet über http://dnb.dnb.de abrufbar.

Herstellung und Verlag: BoD –
Books on Demand, Norderstedt

ISBN: 978-3-7526-4169-1

Introduction

By using this book, you accept this disclaimer in full.

No advice

The book contains information. The information is not advice and should not be treated as such.

No representations or warranties

To the maximum extent permitted by applicable law and subject to section below, we exclude all representations, warranties, undertakings and guarantees relating to the book.

Without prejudice to the generality of the foregoing paragraph, we do not represent, warrant, undertake or guarantee:

- that the information in the book is correct, accurate, complete or non-misleading.

- that the use of the guidance in the book will lead to any particular outcome or result.

Limitations and exclusions of liability

The limitations and exclusions of liability set out in this section and elsewhere in this disclaimer: are subject to section 6 below; and govern all liabilities arising under the disclaimer or in relation to the book, including liabilities arising in contract, in tort (including negligence) and for breach of statutory duty.

We will not be liable to you in respect of any losses arising out of any event or events beyond our reasonable control.

We will not be liable to you in respect of any business losses, including without limitation loss of or damage to profits, income, revenue, use, production, anticipated savings, business, contracts, commercial opportunities or goodwill.

We will not be liable to you in respect of any loss or corruption of any data, database or software.

We will not be liable to you in respect of any special, indirect or consequential loss or damage.

Exceptions

Nothing in this disclaimer shall: limit or exclude our liability for death or personal injury resulting from negligence; limit or exclude our liability for fraud or fraudulent misrepresentation; limit any of our liabilities in any way that is not permitted under applicable law; or exclude any of our liabilities that may not be excluded under applicable law.

Severability

If a section of this disclaimer is determined by any court or other competent authority to be unlawful and/or unenforceable, the other sections of this disclaimer continue in effect.

If any unlawful and/or unenforceable section would be lawful or enforceable if part of it were deleted, that part will be deemed to be deleted, and the rest of the section will continue in effect.

Law and jurisdiction

This disclaimer will be governed by and construed in accordance with Swiss law, and any disputes relating to this disclaimer will be subject to the exclusive jurisdiction of the courts of Switzerland.

Inhaltsverzeichnis

Inhaltsverzeichnis   **9**

Introduction   **11**

Chapter 1: Recipes for People with Kapha Body Type   **12**

Recipe #1- Baked Pears with Kapha Stuffing   *12*

Recipe #2- Multigrain roti   *14*

Recipe #3- Detoxifying Soup   *16*

Recipe #4- Okra with Cumin Seasoning   *18*

Recipe #5- Braised Kale   *19*

Recipe #6- Spiced Lemon Weight Loss Tea   *21*

Recipe #7- Skewed Chicken and Jasmine Rice   *22*

Recipe #8- Smashed Pea and Chicken Sandwiches   *24*

Recipe #9- Cranberry, Carrot and Mushroom Pilaf   *26*

Recipe #10- Apple, Spinach and Couscous with Goat's Cheese   *29*

Chapter 2: Recipes for People with Pitta Body Type   **30**

Recipe #11- Watermelon Sparkle   *30*

Recipe #12- Zucchini Bread   *31*

Recipe #13- Mint and Melon Cooler   *33*

Recipe #14- Crispy Sweet Potato   *35*

Recipe #15- Roasted Brussels Sprout with Honey   *36*

Recipe #16- Fennel Salad Flavored with Fish Sauce   *38*

Recipe #17- Roasted Fennels and Coconut Soup   *40*

Chapter 3: Recipes for People with Vata Body Type   **43**

Recipe #18- Citrus Sweet Potatoes with Cinnamon and Saffron   *43*

Recipe #19- The Special Mung Soup with Veggies   *45*

Recipe #20- Chicken with Oat Crust and Grilled Asparagus
                                                    48

Recipe #21- Mixed Vegetable Soup   *50*

Recipe #22- Chickpea Salad   *52*

Recipe #23- Brown Rice with Buckwheat   *53*

Recipe #24- Chicken with Veggies and Coconut Milk   *55*

Recipe #25- Spicy Almond Milk   *57*

Recipe #26- Coconut Pudding   *58*

Recipe #27- Tasty Carrot Halwa   *60*

Recipe #28- Healthy and Tasty Fried Rice   *61*

Conclusion   **64**

Introduction

This book will teach you how to practice healthy eating following the Ayurvedic principles. Here, I have presented recipes keeping in mind the needs of people with Kapha, Pitta and Vata body types. In spite of abiding by the rules set by Ayurveda and assisting people to reach their ideal body weight, these recipes are highly appetizing. You will love having them regularly. What's more, some of them are sumptuous enough even for being served to guests.

Chapter 1:
Recipes for People with Kapha Body Type

Recipe #1- Baked Pears with Kapha Stuffing

Ingredients

- 8 ripe pears (you shouldn't pick Asian pears)
- ½ cup finely diced dried apricots
- ½ cup pine nuts
- ½ cup orange juice
- A drizzle of honey (you cannot use more as you are cooking for people with kapha body type)
- A drizzle of olive oil (you cannot use more as you are cooking for people with kapha body type)

How to prepare?

1. Set your oven to preheat at 350°. Grease a baking dish using a few drops of olive oil.
2. Cut all the pears into two halves (lengthwise). Remove their seeds and stem, which will leave a petite hollow in each of the halves.
3. Use your food processor to puree the pieces of apricot. Add a part of the orange juice (ideally, you should add 70% of the mentioned amount) to the puree and blend the two ingredients well. The resulting mix should be absolutely smooth.
4. Now, put in the pine nuts.
5. Take a spoonful of the apricot mixture and fill the hollowed pears.
6. Arrange all pear halves (you should have 16) on the greased baking dish. Pour the remaining orange juice over

the stuffed pears and add a drizzle of olive oil.

7. Cover the tray using aluminum foil and put it inside the preheated oven for baking. You should bake the pears for around an hour or until they turn tender.

8. Take the tray out from the oven and allow the pear halves to cool. Once they are lukewarm, drizzle the honey and serve.

Recipe #2- Multigrain roti

Ingredients

- Old wheat
- Sorghum
- Old rice
- Barley seeds
- Horse gram
- Mung bean

How to prepare?

1. Take all the above-mentioned ingredients in equal quantity.
2. Soak them in a bowlful of water overnight (ideally, you should soak these grains for a minimum of 6 hours for getting the desired results).
3. Drain the water and dry the grains. The best way of doing that is spreading all the grains on a newspaper and keeping them under the sun.
4. Place a wide pan over medium to high heat. Once the pan is hot, add the dried grains little by little to it. Once the grains are semi-fried, (they shouldn't turn too dark, but must start releasing aroma), remove them from the pan.

5. Powder the fried grains using a grinder and store it in an airtight container.
6. Use the powder to prepare multi-grain roti.

Recipe #3- Detoxifying Soup

Ingredients

- 8 cups of pure water
- ½ cup of chopped celery
- ½ cup of shredded carrot
- 1 cup of chopped kale
- 12 black peppercorns
- ½ teaspoon turmeric
- 2 teaspoons cumin seeds
- 4 thin slices of fresh ginger
- 1 teaspoon rock salt (it's an optional ingredient)

How to prepare?

1. Take a large pot and put all the ingredients mentioned in the above list. Combine well and place the pot over medium to high heat.
2. Once the mixture starts boiling, reduce the heat. Simmer for around 60 to 90 minutes.
3. Remove the pot from the heat. Use the back of a ladle for mashing the boiled vegetables against the sides of the pot.
4. Strain out the liquid in a bowl. Serve it warm. The solids should be discarded.

Recipe #4- Okra with Cumin Seasoning

Ingredients

- 2 cups of okras (wash them well, soak and dry)
- 1 teaspoon cumin seeds
- ½ teaspoon mustard seeds
- ¼ teaspoon turmeric
- ¼ teaspoon chili powder
- 1 teaspoon olive oil
- Salt to taste

How to prepare?

1. Take two cups of fresh okras and wash them well. Soak the okra in water for some time and get it dried by the time you start cooking.
2. Cut the okras into thick slices.

3. Heat the oil over medium to high heat and fry the sliced okra in it. Once it's almost done, put in the cumin and mustard seeds. Stir for a few seconds and add the chili powder, turmeric and salt. Cook for 2 to 3 more minutes and your okra will be ready to be served. Here, I would like to note that you should never cover the pan when cooking okra. That would turn the vegetable sticky.
4. This okra recipe is a perfect match for multigrain roti.

Recipe #5- Braised Kale

Ingredients

- 4 cups of curly kale (stem, rib and chop the greens)
- Rock salt
- Freshly ground black pepper

- 2 teaspoons chopped parsley
- ¼ teaspoon sweet paprika
- ¼ teaspoon turmeric
- 2 tablespoons olive oil

How to prepare?

1. Place a pan over medium heat and heat the olive oil in it. Put in the black pepper, turmeric and paprika and stir for a few seconds or until the spices start releasing aroma.
2. Put in the chopped kale, add the salt and cover the pan. Reduce heat and cook for around 15 minutes or until the kale becomes tender.
3. Your Braised Kale is now ready. Garnish with the chopped parsley. This dish should also be served hot.

Recipe #6- Spiced Lemon Weight Loss Tea

Ingredients

- 4 drops of apple cider vinegar
- 2 pinches of cayenne pepper (each pinch is equal to 1/6 teaspoon of cayenne pepper)
- 2 teaspoons honey
- ½ lemon
- 2 cups water

How to prepare?

- Boil the water.
- Extract juice from the lemon and add to the boiled water. Also, add the other ingredients mentioned above and stir well. If you don't get apple cider vinegar, you can use any other type of vinegar you prefer.

- The refreshing tea is now ready to be consumed. You can have it every morning in empty stomach, half an hour before each meal or you can even sip the tea slowly after lunch and dinner. Ideally, you should take this tea once or twice every day.

Recipe #7- Skewed Chicken and Jasmine Rice

Ingredients

- 2 cups jasmine rice
- 2 chicken breasts
- 2 teaspoons rice wine vinegar
- 2 tablespoons soy sauce
- 1 teaspoon honey
- ½ cup of diced yellow or red bell pepper
- ½ cup of diced onion
- 4 bamboo skewers (soak them in water for an hour)

How to prepare?

1. Begin by cooking the rice following the instructions printed on the box.

2. As you wait for the rice to get cooked, get the chicken breasts ready. Dice them into square pieces (each should be of 1 inch). Take a large bowl and mix the chicken, bell paper and onions in it. Put in the honey, vinegar and soy sauce. Marinate the chicken for around 30 minutes (if you want, you can marinate for a longer duration).

3. Now, you will have to arrange the ingredients on the bamboo skewers. First insert onion, follow it up with bell pepper and then insert a piece of chicken. Keep repeating in this order until the ingredients cover the entire skewer.

4. Place a nonstick grill pan over medium-low heat and heat the olive oil

in it. Place the skewers and heat for around 10 minutes or until the chicken is duly cooked.
5. Once the chicken is ready, serve it hot with steamed jasmine rice.

Recipe #8- Smashed Pea and Chicken Sandwiches

Ingredients

- 2 cups of shredded chicken
- ½ cup of mashed avocado
- ½ cup of shelled peas
- 4 tablespoons of Greek yogurt
- 2 tablespoons lemon juice
- 1 teaspoon salt
- 1 teaspoon freshly ground black pepper
- 8 slices of thick bread

How to prepare?

1. Your first job would be preparing smashed peas. For that, you will have to put all the peas in boiling water. Blanch them for a few minutes, remove them from water and finally crush using a fork.

2. Now, add a few drops of lemon juice to the crushed peas. Combine the mashed avocado and crushed peas.

3. Now, in a separate bowl, combine the chicken with salt, pepper and yogurt.

4. Take a slice of bread and cover it with a layer of the pea and avocado spread. Next, put some shredded chicken over it. Place another slice of bread over the chicken. Smashed Pea and Chicken Sandwich is now ready to be served. Use the remaining ingredients for preparing more such sandwiches.

Recipe #9- Cranberry, Carrot and Mushroom Pilaf

Ingredients

- 2 cups button mushrooms (slice each piece into two halves)
- 2 cups diced carrots
- 2 onions, diced
- 2 cups red or brown rice
- 4 tablespoons dried cranberries
- 2 teaspoons salt
- 2 teaspoons cumin
- 2 bay leaves
- ½ teaspoon turmeric
- 2 cinnamon sticks (if they are too long, 1 will do)
- 2 teaspoons minced ginger
- 2 teaspoons minced garlic
- 4 tablespoons olive oil

- 8 cups water
- ½ cup chopped mint leaves

How to prepare?

1. Place a pan over high heat and heat the olive oil in it. Put in the bay leaves, cinnamon and cumin. Once they start releasing their flavors, add the garlic and ginger.
2. Stir for around a minute or so and then add the onion. Reduce the heat to medium and wait until the onion becomes translucent. Now, add the button mushrooms. Sauté them for around 3 minutes.
3. Next, put in the carrots. Cook the mix for another five minutes or until the carrots become a bit tender.
4. Reduce the heat to low and add all the remaining spices. Allow the ingredients to simmer for some time.

5. In the mean time, wash the red/brown rice meticulously with water.

6. Put the washed rice into the mix you were preparing. Combine all the ingredients well.

7. Wait for 5 minutes and add the water. Place the lid and cook for around 40 minutes over low heat. You'll have to be careful about the time the rice takes to be cooked properly. It's because the time required tend to vary depending on the type of rice you are using.

8. Garnish the pilaf using mint leaves when serving.

Recipe #10- Apple, Spinach and Couscous with Goat's Cheese

Ingredients

- 2 cups couscous (boil and fluff it)
- 2 cups baby spinach
- 2 medium-sized apples, chopped
- 1 teaspoon black pepper
- 2 teaspoons salt
- 4 tablespoons grated goat's cheese

How to prepare?

1. Combine the baby spinach, apple and couscous. Add freshly ground pepper and salt. Mix all the ingredients well and sprinkle the grated goat's cheese.
2. This item tastes great both when served hot and cold.

Chapter 2:
Recipes for People with Pitta Body Type

Recipe #11- Watermelon Sparkle

Ingredients

- Sparkling water
- 1 small cucumber, peeled cups cubes of watermelon
- Juice extracted from 1 lime
- 5 to 6 fresh mint leaves
- 1 pinch ground cinnamon
- A tiny pinch of pink salt

How to prepare?

1. Take all the ingredients besides sparkling water and puree them in your blender. Continue until you get a smooth mix.
2. Fill 50% of a glass with the watermelon mix you just prepared. Fill the remaining glass with water. Before serving, garnish using a fresh mint leaf.

Recipe #12- Zucchini Bread

Ingredients

- 4 egg whites
- 1 cup olive oil
- 1 cup honey
- 4 cups of grated zucchini
- 4 tsp vanilla extract
- 3 tsp cinnamon

- 2 cups whole wheat flour
- 2 cups spelt flour
- 1 tsp salt
- 1 cup sunflower seeds
- 1 tsp baking soda
- ½ tsp baking powder

How to prepare?

1. Set the oven to preheat at 350°F.
2. Take four bread pans (ideally, they should be 8x4 inch pans). Grease the pans using olive oil.
3. Take a large bowl and put the honey, oil, vanilla essence and egg whites. Combine the ingredients well and put in the zucchini.
4. Take another bowl and in it combine the dry ingredients such as the two types of flour, cinnamon powder, baking soda, baking powder and salt. Mix them together using a spoon or

your hand. There shouldn't be any lump in this dry mix.

5. Now add the dry mix to the egg mix. Combine thoroughly and transfer the batter into the pans.

6. Place the pans into the preheated oven and bake for around an hour. Continue baking until the knife or toothpick inserted into the bread's middle emerges clean.

Recipe #13- Mint and Melon Cooler

Ingredients

- 2 cups water
- 2 cups sugar
- Zest taken from a couple of limes
- A cupful of watermelon cubes
- 2 cups chopped mint

How to prepare?

1. Take a sauce pot and place it over medium heat. Put the water and sugar in and cook until you see the sugar dissolving and the liquid bubbling.
2. Remove the sugar mix from heat and add the lime zest and mint leaves. Allow the mixture to come to room temperature.
3. Once it cools down, strain the minty sugar syrup. Transfer it into a lidded container and refrigerate.
4. Prepare melon juice by blending the water melon cubes in your food processor.
5. Once the syrup is perfectly cold, combine ¼ cup of the syrup with the lemon juice. Stir well, put into a tall glass and serve after garnishing the drink with a fresh mint leaf.

Recipe #14- Crispy Sweet Potato

Ingredients

- 5 small sweet potatoes (slice them)
- 3 tbsp olive oil
- 1 tsp ground cinnamon
- 1 tsp rock salt
- ½ tsp paprika or cayenne pepper

How to prepare?

1. Set the oven to preheat at 400 degrees.
2. In a bowl, combine all the above mentioned seasonings with the olive oil.
3. Put the potato slices into the oil-mix. Toss meticulously so that each slice gets properly coated.
4. Take a baking sheet (ungreased) and line the coated slices of sweet

potatoes on it. You can also use a sheet of parchment paper.

5. Transfer the lined baking sheet into the preheated oven. Bake the potatoes for around 10 minutes. Turn the potato slices and bake for another 10 minutes. Both sides should turn golden brown.

6. Serve the crispy sweet potatoes hot.

Recipe #15- Roasted Brussels Sprout with Honey

Ingredients

- 3 lb Brussels sprouts
- ½ cup of olive oil
- ½ tsp black pepper (freshly ground)
- 1 tsp seal salt
- 4 tbsp honey
- ½ cup of sunflower seeds, toasted
- ½ cup of pepitas (toasted)

How to prepare?

1. Set the oven to preheat at 375°F.
2. Rinse the Brussels sprouts carefully. Make sure that all the discolored or brown outer leaves have been removed. Cut their stems off and slice them into halves.
3. Take a large bowl and in it toss the halved Brussels sprouts using olive oil. Also, add black pepper and salt.
4. After coating the Brussels sprouts evenly with the ingredients mentioned above, spread them into a baking sheet (it should be lined with parchment paper).
5. Place the sheet into the oven and roast for 15 minutes. Stir the sprouts using a spatula and roast for another 30 minutes. Now, put some honey over them. Stir thoroughly to coat.
6. Roast for another 15 minutes. Stop roasting only when you are confident

that the Brussels sprouts have become fork tender.

7. Serve the Brussels sprouts after mixing them with pepitas and sunflower
seeds.

Recipe #16- Fennel Salad Fla-vored with Fish Sauce

Ingredients

For the fennel mix

- 2 fennel bulbs (keep the fronds), chopped into ¼ inch pieces
- 2 small carrots (peel and chop them finely)
- ½ cup of chopped green and purple cab-bage

For the dressing

- 2 tsp sesame or sunflower seeds
- 2 tsp fish sauce
- 2 tsp sesame oil
- 1 tbsp apple cider vinegar
- 1 tbsp sunflower oil
- 4 cloves minced garlic
- 1 tbsp finely chopped scallion
- 2 tsp dried mint
- ½ tsp red pepper flakes

How to prepare?

1. Chop the fennel bulbs (also chop the talks and fronds) into ¼ inch pieces. Chop enough cabbage (both green and purple) for filling half a cup. Peel the carrots and chop them finely. All these ingredients should be kept in a large bowl. Set the bowl aside and move to the next step.

2. Mix the sesame seeds, sesame oil, fish sauce, apple cider vinegar, dried mint and sunflower oil together in a mixing bowl.
3. Drizzle the olive oil dressing over the chopped ingredients and begin tossing. Continue until all the ingredients are coated perfectly with the olive oil dressing. The salad is now ready to be served.

Recipe #17- Roasted Fennels and Coconut Soup

Ingredients

- 4 fennel bulbs (you should cut them lengthwise into ½ inch thick pieces)
- 10 large carrots (peel them and cut them into 1.2 inch cubes)
- 4 leeks (remove the tops, clean thoroughly and cut them into halves)

- 2 cups coconut milk
- 2 cups vegetable broth
- 4 tbsp olive oil
- 2 tbsp coriander powder
- 3 tsp cumin seeds
- 2 tsp agave nectar
- Sea salt to taste

How to prepare?

1. Set the oven to preheat at 400°F.
2. Arrange the leeks, fennel and carrots on greased (grease with olive oil) baking sheets. Season using sea salt, coriander and cumin. Bake for around 40 minutes or until you see the items turning light brown.
3. Transfer the baked veggies into your food processor. Add the vegetable broth and coconut milk and switch on the food processor. Blend until you get a smooth puree. Divide the soup into bowls, garnish using

toasted pecans and fennel fronds and serve. You can also top the soup with some shredded coconut.

Chapter 3:
Recipes for People with Vata Body Type

Recipe #18- Citrus Sweet Potatoes with Cinnamon and Saffron

Ingredients

- 2 sweet potatoes (cut them into ½ inch cubes)
- 1 white onion, finely chopped
- 2 tablespoons coconut oil
- ½ cup coconut milk (try to use freshly extracted coconut milk)
- Zest taken from 1 orange
- 2 teaspoons cinnamon
- ½ teaspoon nutmeg
- 2 teaspoons ginger powder
- 1/8 teaspoon saffron

- Sea salt to taste

How to prepare?

1. Place a sauce pan over medium heat and heat the coconut oil in it. Put in the onions, ginger powder, nutmeg and cinnamon. Sauté the ingredients for 3 to 4 minutes or until you see the onions turn translucent.
2. Now, add the coconut milk, orange zest, saffron and cubes of sweet potato. Place the lid, reduce the heat and simmer for 12 to 15 minutes. Don't forget to stir the mix occasionally. If you don't do so, the mixture might get stuck to the pan's bottom.
3. Once you are sure that the sweet potato has been properly cooked, remove the pan from heat. Mash the potatoes roughly (you'll not need pureed potato for preparing this dish).

4. Add salt. Serve the dish with blanched veggies.

Recipe #19- The Special Mung Soup with Veggies

Ingredients:

- 2 cups split mung lentil
- 16 cups water
- 4 cups sliced summer squash (each slice should be of around ½ inch)
- 2 cups sliced carrots (each slice should be of around ½ inch)
- 2 teaspoons coriander powder
- ½ teaspoon asafetida
- Lemon juice to taste
- 4 tablespoons clarified butter
- ½ teaspoon turmeric
- 2 teaspoons sea salt
- 1 teaspoon freshly minced ginger

- 1 green capsicum, finely chopped
- 2 tablespoons black mustard seeds
- 1 teaspoon cumin seeds

How to prepare?

1. In a pan, heat the clarified butter (if you are not fond of clarified butter, you can use your favorite cooking oil).
2. To it, add the cumin seeds and asafetida. Once the cumin seeds stop sputtering, add all spices mentioned above and two tablespoons of water. Sauté the ingredients for around 30 seconds (the heat should be kept low). Don't overdo sautéing as that might burn your spices.
3. Put in the beans. Sauté for another 2 minutes. Now add all the chopped veggies. Heat for 2 more minutes. Keep stirring to ensure all the

ingredients blend perfectly with each other.

4. Add the ginger, pepper, salt, and some water. Increase the heat and wait until the mixture starts boiling. Again reduce the heat to medium-low, cover the pan and allow the mix to cook for around 45 minutes.

5. To another pan, add some clarified butter, mustard seeds and cumin seeds. Once the seeds start popping, add them to the lentil soup (along with the clarified butter).

6. Remove the soup from heat and divide it into bowls. Garnish with chopped coriander and serve.

Recipe #20- Chicken with Oat Crust and Grilled Asparagus

Ingredients

- 4 chicken breasts (thin them out using meat pallet)
- 1 cup oats (opt for the variety that cooks quickly)
- 1 cup regular bread crumbs
- 2 fresh basil leaves
- 1 teaspoon rock salt
- ½ cup flour
- 8 tablespoons olive oil
- 2 eggs (whisk it in a bowl)
- 3 cloves of garlic, crushed
- 1 bunch asparagus

How to prepare?

1. In a wide plate, mix the bread crumbs, oats and basil leaves.

2. Place a non stick pan over medium heat and heat the olive oil in it.
3. Spread the flour on a plate. Place the bowl with the whisked eggs and the plate with the flour beside each other.
4. Take a chicken breast and coat it evenly with flour. Dip it into the beaten egg and coat again with the bread crumb-oat mix.
5. Place the chicken breast into the hot oil and cook for 5 to 7 minutes. Turn and cook the other side for another 5 to 7 minutes. You should ideally cook the chicken breast until both its sides turn crisp and golden.
6. Take a non-stick grill pan and grease it thoroughly using olive oil. Add the asparagus and garlic. Cook them (over medium heat) for 5 minutes.
7. Top the chicken breasts with the grilled garlic and asparagus and serve hot.

Recipe #21- Mixed Vegetable Soup

(although I am including this in recipes meant for people with Vata body type, it can be had by Pitta and Kapha people too)

Ingredients

- 4 cups vegetables (as this is for Vata people, opt for carrots, for Pitta and Kapha people I would recommend mixed seasonal vegetables)
- 8 cups water
- 6 peppercorns
- 1 teaspoon cumin seeds
- 10 cardamom pods
- 10 cloves
- An 1 inch stick of cinnamon
- 2 tablespoons clarified butter
- Salt to taste

How to prepare?

1. Cut the carrots into 1 inch pieces.
2. Place a pot over medium heat and cook the carrot in it until the pieces turn tender.
3. Grind peppercorn, cardamom, cinnamon, cumin seeds and cloves either using your blender or mortar and pestle.
4. Place a large saucepan over medium to high heat and add the clarified butter to it. Put in all the ground spices and sauté for a few seconds. You should do this carefully to ensure that your spices don't burn.
5. Now, add the carrots and the water you sued for cooking the carrots. Bring the mixture to boil. Wait for two minutes and add salt. Serve the soup hot.

Ingredients

- 1 cup uncooked chickpeas (soak them in warm water overnight and boil them the next morning)
- 2 large tomatoes, finely chopped
- 2 large cucumbers, finely chopped
- 2 mangoes, finely chopped (you can also use avocados, apples or peaches)
- ½ teaspoon salt
- 2 tablespoons honey
- 2 tablespoons olive oil
- 2 teaspoons apple cider vinegar
- 2 fresh basil leaves

How to prepare?

1. In a mixing bowl, combine the apple cider vinegar, honey, olive oil, basil leaves and salt. Blend the ingredients

well and add the boiled chickpeas.
Mix and put in all the chopped veggies.

2. Mix all ingredients together. The
   salad is now ready to be served.
   Serve it hot with a drizzle of lime
   juice.

Recipe #23- Brown Rice with Buckwheat

Ingredients

- 1 cup of buckwheat
- 1 cup of brown rice
- 8 cups water (you might need to use a bit more or a bit less water for getting the desired thickness)
- ½ teaspoon mineral salt
- ⅓ teaspoon turmeric
- ½ teaspoon freshly grated ginger (you can also use black pepper instead)

- 4 tablespoons clarified butter
- ½ teaspoon mineral salt
- ½ cup of chopped cashews

How to prepare?

1. Put all the ingredients barring the clarified butter and cashews inside a pot and place it over medium to high heat.
2. Once the water starts boiling, reduce the heat and simmer the mix for around 45 minutes. If you are looking for faster results, you can cook in a pressure cooker; the ingredients will be ready in just 18 minutes when cooked at pressure.
3. Once the cooking is done, stir the mixture a few times and remove it from heat. Allow it to sit for five minutes.
4. In the mean time, heat the clarified butter in a saucepan over low heat.

Sauté the cashews in it for 5 to 7 minutes or until the nuts start releasing aroma. Stir in the cashews and the clarified butter into the porridge and serve the dish hot.

Recipe #24- Chicken with Veggies and Coconut Milk

Ingredients

- 4 chicken breast (cut them into ½ inch thick pieces)
- ½ cup vegetable or chicken stock
- 2 cups coconut milk
- 8 cloves of garlic, minced
- 2 one inch blocks of ginger, finely chopped
- 2 large carrots, diced
- 2 large onions, diced
- 2 teaspoons paprika
- 2 teaspoons black pepper

- 2 teaspoons salt
- 6 teaspoons olive oil

How to prepare?

1. Place a pan over medium to high heat and heat olive oil in it. Put the ginger and garlic in and wait for them to become translucent. Put in the onion. Cook until they turn light brown.

2. Add the diced carrots. Cook until they become soft.

3. Put in the spices, chicken/vegetable stock, and coconut milk. Stir the ingredients together and add the chicken slices.

4. Reduce the heat and simmer for 10 minutes (at times, you may need to cook a few minutes more for the chicken to be ready). You may add some more water if you want the sauce to have lighter consistency.

5. Once the chicken is perfectly cooked, remove the pan from heat and

transfer the chicken and the sauce into a serving plate. Garnish with chopped chives or parsley and serve. This item tastes best when eaten with breads and rice.

Recipe #25- Spicy Almond Milk

Ingredients

- A cup of almonds
- 2 cups water
- ¼ teaspoon ginger powder
- ¼ teaspoon cardamom powder
- ¼ teaspoon cinnamon powder

How to prepare?

1. Soak the almond in water overnight. For best results, you should soak the nuts in water for at least 7 to 8 hours.

2. The next day, peel off the skin of your almonds.
3. Now, blend the soaked almond in your blender with 2 cups water.
4. Use a sieve or a muslin cloth for straining the freshly prepared almond milk.
5. You can drink the almond milk like that or can spice it up a bit by adding freshly ground spices such as cardamom, cinnamon and ginger.

Recipe #26- Coconut Pudding

Ingredients

- 2 tablespoons clarified butter
- 100 grams jaggery
- 200 grams desiccated coconut
- 400 ml freshly extracted coconut milk
- 500 ml soya milk
- 1 teaspoon cinnamon powder

- 2 teaspoons rosewater
- 6 heaped tablespoons rice flour
- 1/2 teaspoon cardamom powder

How to prepare?

1. Soak the desiccated coconut in very little water.
2. Heat the clarified butter and jaggery in a pan over medium to high heat until the jaggery starts melting.
3. Put in the soaked coconut, soya milk, coconut milk and all the spices.
4. Let the mixture to boil. Once it starts boiling, slowly add the rice flour. Keep beating using a whisk to prevent formation of lumps. Stir for 3 to 4 more minutes.
5. Pour the mixture into a bowl. Transfer the bowl into the refrigerator to allow the pudding to set for a couple of hours. Serve your Coconut Pudding cold (it shouldn't be too cold).

Recipe #27- Tasty Carrot Halwa

Ingredients

- 6 carrots
- 8 pods of cardamom (you'll have to grind them before using)
- ½ teaspoon cinnamon powder
- 4 tablespoons ground almonds (you can also use desiccated coconut)
- Water
- Clarified butter
- Jaggery
- ½ cup soya milk

How to prepare?

1. Grate the carrots as finely as possible. Thick grating will not give you the desired results.

2. You will have to decide how much water, jaggery and clarified butter you'll use depending on your preferences.
3. Place a saucepan over medium heat and put the grated carrots into it.
4. Put in all the remaining ingredients barring the soy milk into the pan. Reduce the heat and simmer for around 20 minutes. Ideally, you should continue until the carrots become tender.
5. Now, add the soy milk. Stir for another 5 to 7 minutes and your halwa will be ready. Serve it hot after garnishing with some sliced almonds.

Recipe #28- Healthy and Tasty Fried Rice

Ingredients

- One cup of mixed vegetables (pick broccoli, carrots and cabbage)
- ½ tsp cumin powder
- ½ tsp turmeric powder
- ½ tsp ground coriander
- ½ teaspoon cardamom powder
- 1 tablespoon clarified butter (if you are making it for a Vata person, you can use some more clarified butter)
- Salt to taste

How to prepare?

1. Boil the vegetables.
2. Cook the rice.
3. Place a pot over medium heat, and add the clarified butter. Once it starts melting, add the turmeric powder, cumin powder and ground coriander.
4. Sauté the spices for a few minutes and put in the veggies. Add the cardamom powder and salt. Mix well.

5. Finally add the cooked rice. Mix all the ingredients meticulously and serve hot.

Conclusion

This cookbook has recipes that are easy to prepare, nutritious, and amazingly tasty. Try them out at home and see yourself getting healthier following the parameters set by Ayurveda.